OVERCOMING OVERTHINKING & RUMINATION

40 techniques to stop overthinking and rumination, relieve stress, stop negativity, and declutter your mind.

James C. Clever

Copyright©2022 James E. Clever

All Rights Reserved

INTRODUCTION

Overthinking is a restless propensity that being experience frequently in psychotherapy practice. There are numerous ways people tend to overthink, for example, repeating the past — replaying a similar situation again and again in one's mind. Worrying is another type, where we fixate on what the future could bring.

We are gifted with a brain that, generally, is a wondrous creation that empowers us to handle information, thoroughly consider our choices, and decide how to continue.

In any case, on occasion, our psyches can seem like the cause of all our problems. At the point when we find ourselves overthinking an issue, with our viewpoints returning over and over to a past circumstance or future situation, we're probably going to unnecessarily break ourselves down.

Consistent worrying and overthinking can frequently prompt issues with psychological wellness, peace, and prosperity. Procedures like profound breathing, reflection, self-empathy, and requesting help from a medical services proficient can assist with lightening the pressure of overthinking.

Damaging idea designs

You at long last have a couple of calm minutes to yourself, just to promptly begin contemplating whether you neglected to send that thank-you email or whether you've misjudged your possibilities of getting the promotion or advancement.

Sound natural? Worrying and overthinking is essential for the human experience, however, when left uncontrolled, they can negatively affect your health and well-being. Harping on similar contemplations might try and build your risk of specific psychological well-being conditions.

Thus, it's to our greatest advantage to stop this overthinking propensity from really developing and this book is written to give your assistance in stopping or overcoming overthinking and rumination.

James C. Clever

CHAPTER ONE

WHAT IS OVERTHINKING?

Everyone worries occasionally - so while does worry becomes overthinking?

Overthinking basically as the name proposes - thinking excessively. Overthinking is rehashing a similar idea to excess, breaking down the least complex of circumstances or occasions until all feeling of extent has gone. The overthinking mind can't make an interpretation of these contemplations into activities or good results or provide solutions, so thusly makes sensations of worry, stress, anxiety, and tension.

Has anybody at any time pointed out, "you are overthinking"? You're in good company. A large number of us know all about the experience of overthinking, regardless of whether we haven't characterized it thusly. By and large, "overthinking" alludes to the course of dreary, ineffective ideas. Since contemplations can be centered around various things, research has commonly separated between "rumination" over a significant time, and "stress" about what's in store. Notwithstanding which word we use, we are discussing consistent idea circles that don't appear to have a goal.

Your capacity to believe is one of your most noteworthy gifts as an individual. Our cerebrums have advanced to create complex considerations that permit us to figure out information, tackle issues, prepare, and gain from before. As a result of thinking, we have created complex and beautiful societies and developed wonderful innovations over time.

Be that as it may, the well-established proverb "an overdose of something that is otherwise good" strikes a chord here. At the point when we overthink, stress, or ruminate, we are positively thinking. The separation of "over"- thinking features that our reasoning isn't getting us anyplace and isn't useful to us. So assuming you notice that you are stuck contemplating a similar issue again and again but are not coming to any kind of solution but are just being disturbed you might be overthinking.

Certainly, we as a whole overthink somewhat? As guardians, children or girls, workers or finance managers, stressing over things is connected to thinking often about our friends and family, and about working effectively.

Notwithstanding, individuals who truly battle with overthinking will more often than not be "ruminators", going over occasions that have proactively occurred. Regular worrying will in general be over what's in store: could I at any point fulfill this time constraint? Might I at any point track down a decent private level for my mum? Frequently, our concerns assist us with moving advances as we are sorting out how to alleviate them; but overthinking will in general be latent as opposed to dynamic, harping on previous occasions and developing lopsidedly bad future outcomes.

It's the primitive emotional part of your brain that overthinking comes from. In the same way as other characteristics of tension and gloom, overthinking really comes from one of our crude safeguarding senses.

The crude psyche will continuously see things from the absolute worst viewpoint. This is because the brain is being hyper-careful, attempting to keep us alive - there's no sense in being hopeful about those saber-toothed tigers I've referenced previously!

The scholarly cerebrum will let us know that not a chance will we lose our employment since we called our manager by some unacceptable name. Notwithstanding, individuals inclined to rumination are answering in that crude survival mode, where zeroing in on the most pessimistic scenario situations is bound to keep us alive.

Overthinking and uneasiness cooperate, intensifying the sensations of stress and vulnerability.

WHAT CAUSES OVERTHINKING?

At its root, overthinking is a programmed self-security system. What do you tend to overthink? There is the possibility is that your focus is on funds, wellbeing, work, connections, and significance. Feeling in charge of these various spaces can bear the cost of a feeling of prosperity and, obviously, you need the best for yourself. Notwithstanding, the key here is that pondering these regions in a useless manner does practically nothing to further develop them.

We don't overthink intentionally. Contemplations are most frequently programmed and constant, implying that overthinking turns into a propensity - we don't rest around evening time or sit in the morning and contemplate internally; "alright it's time to ruminate for the following two hours." Your mind basically does what it has done before.

CHAPTER TWO

40 TECHNIQUES TO OVERCOME OVERTHINKING

All in all, what's an overthinking individual to do? These tips can assist you with moving in the correct direction.

POSITIVE RETHINKING

This is frequently mistaken for " toxic positivity," which requests that individuals think decidedly — regardless of how troublesome a circumstance is.

Positive rethinking, then again, permits you to recognize the negative viewpoints, then, at that point, requests that you assess whether there's one more method for pondering the circumstance. Maybe there are advantages or things you can change about it.

Example:

You continually regard yourself as grumbling: "I disdain to be a chief. On top of this multitude of cutoff times and obligations, it's difficult to oversee such countless complex characters. It's genuinely and intellectually debilitating. My work simply sucks."

Venting could feel better briefly, however it settles nothing. Also, you'll probably keep on harping on the amount you disdain your work or how awful you assume you are at making due.

To rehearse good reexamining, supplant the idea above with: "Things are testing at present and I'm feeling disengaged from certain things on my plate. I keep thinking about whether I can transform anything about this present circumstance or my assumptions regarding it."

This thought design enables you to change what is happening. You could begin a little by looking at what significant undertakings need to finish first, then either deferral or agent the rest until you are feeling less restless. The key is to make a stride back and manage things each in turn.

WRITE DOWN YOUR VIEWPOINTS ONCE, THEN OCCUPY YOURSELF FOR 24 HOURS

At the point when our minds think we are in struggle or peril, an underlying caution framework goes off inside to safeguard us.

One thing I have made progress with is recording my sentiments and holding up no less than 24 hours (or only a couple of hours in the event that it's a critical matter) prior to answering or making any kind of hasty move.

Then, I set that draft aside while I divert myself to another undertaking.

Example:

You just got an email about something that turned out badly. You are vexed, your heart begins to race, your breathing gets shallow, and you become hyper-zeroed in on what's turning out badly and why it's your shortcoming.

In the event that you answer the email while your cerebrum is in "caution mode," you could make statements you'll lament later on, which may then fuel the endless loop of overthinking.

Recording negative considerations remove the power from them; I frequently don't want to make a move in view of my fears whenever I've thought of them down.

PRACTICE 'EXPLICIT APPRECIATION'

It's hard to be overpowered by stress while we're remembering our good fortune. Consistently, make a rundown of five things for which you're grateful. Attempt to shift your message down, so you're not consequently writing down similar things. Think about imparting your rundown to a companion, so you can urge each other to look on the splendid side.

In brain science, we know that offering thanks can expand our bliss. It can help us contextualize our dissatisfactions against what we love and assist us with interfacing with an option that could be bigger than ourselves — whether that is others, creatures, nature, or a higher power.

Yet, I find that rehashing a similar appreciation practice, again and again, can become repetition and decrease the profits. For my purposes, it can begin to feel like an insignificant task rather than a careful practice. Along these lines, I like to work on something that I call "explicit appreciation."

Example:

Rather than writing in my diary each day that "I am appreciative for my wellbeing," I'll compose something like, "I'm thankful that I awakened today with no back aggravation and can do the present exercise."

This assists me with keeping fixed on the present time and place, instead of overthinking general deliberations. Tomorrow, I could in any case be appreciative for my wellbeing, yet I could explicitly be thankful that I have sufficient energy for the long run.

AWARENESS

To start with, notice when you're overthinking. At the point when you feel restless, distinguish what your psyche is doing. Could it be said that you are going, again and again, something in your mind? Could it be said that one is thought tediously twirling around in your cerebrum, without your gaining any headway or coming to any goal regarding this situation? That is overthinking.

COUNT THE EXPENSE

Perceive that your overthinking is causing you more damage than great. In some cases, we trust that in the event that we simply consider an issue for quite some time, we'll have the option to sort out an answer. Nonetheless, there comes a moment when our monotonous examination can perplex us, unleash destruction with our rest (which can disable our reasoning), impede our imagination, and disrupt our seeing and valuing of the present (prompting our later lament of having passed up significant subtleties), and channel our energy, any of which can cause loss of motion. Different aftereffects of overthinking can include: secluding ourselves from individuals and circumstances we dread that might make us self-conscious, utilizing liquor, medications, or gorging to numb our sentiments or stop our unremitting contemplations. It's not worth the effort.

CONSIDER WHAT COULD GO RIGHT, AS OPPOSED TO WHAT COULD TURN OUT BADLY.

The main choice induces trust and excitement, though the subsequent choice varieties dread and despondency. Why not utilize your brain in a useful manner, on the off chance that you wind up considering what is going on? In any event, while thinking decidedly, however, it's best not to overthink things and on second thought pass on the outcomes to work out as they may (besides doing your part - and just your part).

GET DEALING WITH THIS ASAP.

With time, overthinking can turn into a profoundly instilled propensity. The more we think in a specific way, the more grounded that brain connection in our cerebrum becomes. It's like strolling along a specific way in the forest. Continuously the way turns out to be progressively very much worn, while the foliage encompassing the way keeps on developing, so it becomes simpler to pick the natural way and more challenging to manufacture an alternate street. Thus, the sooner you do whatever it may take to bring an end to the overthinking propensity, the better.

DISTRACT YOURSELF

Distract yourself with solid, sustaining exercises, like playing with your pet, talking with a companion (about subjects other than the object of your ongoing fixation), working out, reflecting, a decent book, and so forth. Brief interruption can work on your temperament, offer your psyche a reprieve, and permit you to return later to the main thing with new, inventive approaches to adapting to the circumstance.

FOCUS ON TAKING THE FOLLOWING, BEST, SMART ACTIVITY, AS PER YOUR BEST ASSURANCE.

Rather than allowing your psyche to stay in a spiral about envisioned future situations, utilize your energy beneficially. Compose that email, clean your office or kitchen for 15 minutes, or basically shut your eyes and inhale gradually and profoundly for a couple of seconds. Ask yourself, "what might an individual who loves and regards herself/himself really do at the present time?", and act as needs are. Frequently essentially making a move can ease the uneasiness and fixating, while latent fixating simply intensifies the issue.

WRITE OUT ELECTIVE CLARIFICATIONS AND OPPORTUNITIES FOR YOUR CIRCUMSTANCE AND WORRIES.

Suppose that you at first recorded on paper, "I'm alarmed that my exhibition audit at my specific employment will go ineffectively, and I'll be terminated." You can then list things you've done well in your ongoing situation as well as how you've really gained from stumbles you've made at work. The last option can go quite far towards reexamining any missteps on your part (and we as a whole make them), which could prompt a useful conversation during your survey if the matter comes up.

GET SOME PSYCHOLOGICAL AND PROFOUND SEPARATION FROM THE ISSUE.

Imagine that a dear companion of yours, as opposed to you, is battling with the issue. What useful tidbits could you give them? Frequently when we move away from a circumstance, we can see things all the more obviously and equitably and are less genuinely responsive.

IMAGINE A STOP SIGN.

Assuming you find your psyche entangled in mental fixation, picture a STOP sign and tell yourself "Stop!", or even hold up your hand and say "Stop!" In doing as such, you'll foster a new, more useful propensity for (benevolent) letting yourself know that that's it, and guiding your focus toward additional useful pursuits.

USE THE STOP ABBREVIATION TO REMIND YOURSELF TO

1. Stop
2. Take a breath,
3. Observe what's happening inside and around you, and
4. Proceed with the following demonstrated step.

This can assist with zeroing in you on the basics and letting go of unessential considerations that take steps to crash you.

KNOW WHEN YOU'RE ESPECIALLY POWERLESS AGAINST OVER-THE-TOP AND NEGATIVE REASONING

Know when you're especially powerless against over-the-top and negative reasoning and attempt to cease considering an issue/the past/the future at these times.

At the end of the day, be careful HALT (which represents being either Hungry, Angry, Lonely, or Tired). If you're in at least one of these states, your capacity to think plainly and process feelings actually will be impeded. You're likewise bound to succumb to antagonism. Try not to set yourself here. Doing how you want to get back in balance, for example, getting a decent night's rest or eating a good dinner, ought to be your main concern right now.

STOP UTILIZING THE PAST TO ANTICIPATE WHAT'S TO COME.

Since you committed an error or missed the mark concerning your assumptions previously, it doesn't imply that you're ill-fated to bomb the sometime in the not-so-distant future. Apparently, you've acquired some accommodating self-information from your experience, which you can use for your potential benefit from now on.

KEEP COMPANY WITH INDIVIDUALS WHO DON'T OVERTHINK THINGS.

It's been said that we become like the five individuals with whom we invest the most energy. Who are these individuals in your day-to-day existence? Would you like to "get" their perspectives? Since perspectives are for sure infectious.

REMIND YOURSELF WHERE YOU ARE AT THIS MOMENT.

Intellectually or resoundingly, tell yourself, "I'm doing the dishes", "I'm washing up", "I'm taking care of my feline", or regardless. Ground yourself in your current reality. Make this second the focal point of your consideration. This will save you such a lot of mental and close-to-home energy, rather than permitting your brain to veer off into yesterday or tomorrow.

UPDATES YOURSELF WITH THE PRESENT AND REMAIN CALM

Post updates around you to remain present and quiet, for example, "Keep it straightforward", "Each thing in turn", or "Leave it alone". An item, for example, a jewel stone, little stone, or another article that you partner with tranquility, and which you put in no time flat zeroing in on, can likewise assist with bringing you back into the second and into harmony.

REMEMBER YOUR NEEDS AND YOUR PRIORITIES RIGHT.

How does the object of your concern squeeze into the more stupendous plan of your life? Is it actually that significant? Is it safe to say that you are permitting a little issue to create a major shaded area? Is it more significant than your true serenity, wellbeing, and joy? Since, no doubt about it, you are undermining every one of the three assuming you keep on fixating. Therefore, do the first things first.

SET A CUTOFF ON THE TIME IT TAKES YOU TO GO WITH A CHOICE.

At the point when we hesitate on a decision, we can break ourselves down, pass up other significant parts of life, and make things more muddled than they must be. Indeed, unquestionably we might have to get some margin to assemble significant information, yet frequently the most fitting response is not too far off before our nose - we simply get enveloped with attempting to do this "impeccably" (as though something like this existed) or in attempting to stay away from the work or awkward sentiments we may be in for once we really settle on our choice.

For somewhat straightforward choices, set a clock for 15 minutes, gauge your choices, and think of the best (noticeably flawed!) choice, then follow up on it. For additional muddled choices, set a clock for 30 minutes per day (probably) to ponder the matter, then, at that point, redirect the conversation. Assuming you feel enticed to think about the issue over some more, advise yourself that your oblivious mind is working in the background for your sake and that you can continue your critical thinking tomorrow (at the earliest).

TAKE A BREAK FROM THE NEWS AND SOCIAL MEDIA.

Set a breaking point on how frequently you really look at the news, Twitter, Facebook, Instagram, and other media sources.

Besieging your brain with yet more information when you as of now battle with overthinking will simply stoke the fire. Regard the power and clearness of quietness.

For example, you could restrict your media time to 15 minutes three or four times each day.

TAKE A BREAK DURING THE DAY TO BE CLAM

Take standard breaks over the course of the day to accomplish something quiet. This will diminish the possibilities that strain and nervousness will develop inside you and subsequently decrease the probability of your floating into overthinking.

LEARN NEW THINGS.

Learn a genuinely new thing. Take up another dialect, take another yoga class, stroll in another area, or do a crossword puzzle. Channel your psychological energy into something intriguing and inventive.

KNOW YOUR STATE WHETHER IT'S DEPRESSION OR ANXIETY

Consider whether you might be experiencing discouragement or tension. Overthinking is frequently (albeit not generally) an indication of mindset problems. Likewise, overthinking can impede your emotional wellness, so it's an endless loop. You might profit from a guiding meeting with a specialist to address what might be fundamental to your bustling mind.

KNOW THE CONTRAST BETWEEN OVERTHINKING AND CRITICAL THINKING.

There is a period, spot, and approach to consider an issue beneficially. Overthinking centers around the issue. Critical thinking centers around the arrangement, what you've gained from your experience, and your reasonable choices/what you can do now.

PRACTICE REVOLUTIONARY ACKNOWLEDGMENT.

This implies tolerating all parts of your circumstance, including your considerations and your sentiments about your situation. You dislike not having the responses as a whole. You might have an uncomfortable outlook on having committed an error or humiliated yourself. You might feel irate that another person didn't act as per your inclinations. So be it. No different either way, you can acknowledge such is life (or was, assuming that you're thinking about the past). Opposition is pointless (and depleting). The opposition will simply create seriously languishing. Seeing yourself and the circumstance as they truly are will permit you to pull together your consideration on what you can make a move on at this point.

STEP BACK AND SEE HOW YOU'RE ANSWERING

The manner in which you answer your considerations can some of the time keep you in a pattern of rumination, or dull reasoning. Rumination can frequently be on grounds that pessimistic outcomes Trusted Source of an individual's emotional wellness.

The following time you wind up persistently running things over to you, observe what it means for your state of mind. Do you feel disturbed, apprehensive, or blameworthy? What's the essential feeling behind your viewpoints? Having mindfulness is vital to altering your mentality.

FIND AN INTERRUPTION

Close down overthinking by including yourself in an action you appreciate.

This appears to be unique for everybody, except thoughts include:

1. Mastering some new kitchen abilities by handling another recipe
2. Going to your exercise class
3. Taking up another leisure activity, like composition

chipping in with a nearby association

It may be difficult to begin something new when you're overpowered by your thoughts. If finding an interruption feels overwhelming, have a go at saving a little lump of time — say, 30 minutes — each and every other day. Utilize this opportunity to either search for possible interruptions or fiddle with existing ones.

TAKE A FULL BREATH

You've heard it multiple times, yet that is on the grounds that it works. The following time you wind up thrashing around over your viewpoints, shut your eyes and inhale profoundly.

Attempt it

Here is a decent starter exercise to assist you with loosening up with your breath:

1. Track down an agreeable spot to sit and loosen up your neck and shoulders.
2. Place one hand over your heart and the other across your midsection.
3. Breathe in and breathe out through your nose, focusing on how your chest and stomach move as you relax.

Take a stab at doing this exercise 3 times each day for 5 minutes, or at whatever point you have hustling considerations.

MEDITATE

Fostering a standard reflection practice is a proof upheld method for aiding clear your psyche of anxious chat by turning your consideration internal.

All you really want is 5 minutes and a calm spot.

LOOK AT THE MASTER PLAN

How might every one of the issues drifting around to you influence you 5 or 10 years from now? Will anybody truly care that you purchased a natural product plate for the potluck as opposed to baking a pie without any preparation?

Try not to allow minor issues to transform into huge obstacles.

DO SOMETHING DECENT FOR ANOTHER PERSON

Attempting to facilitate the heap for another person can assist you with placing things in context. Consider ways you can help out somebody going through a troublesome time.

Does your companion who's in a separation need a couple of long stretches of youngster care? Might you at any point get food for your neighbor who's been debilitated?

Acknowledging you have the ability to fill somebody's heart with joy better can hold negative considerations back from dominating. It additionally gives you something useful to zero in on rather than your endless stream of considerations.

34.   Recognize programmed negative contemplations (PNCs)

Programmed negative contemplations ((PNCs) allude to automatic negative considerations, as a rule including dread or outrage, which some of the time have in response to a circumstance.

Handling PNCs

You can distinguish and deal with your PNCs by tracking your considerations and effectively attempting to change them:

- Utilize a notebook or notepad to follow what is going on giving you tension, your mindset, and the primary idea that comes to you naturally.

- As you dive into subtleties, assess why the circumstance is causing these negative contemplations.

- Separate the feelings you're encountering and attempt to distinguish what you're enlightening yourself regarding going on.

- Track down an option in contrast to your unique idea. For instance, rather than bouncing directly to, "This will be a legendary disappointment," take a stab at something as per, "I'm truly making an honest effort."

ACKNOWLEDGE YOUR VICTORIES

At the point when you're amidst overthinking, pause and take out your journal or your number one note-taking application on your telephone. Write down five things that have gone directly over the course of the last week and your part in them.

These needn't bother with to be immense achievements. Perhaps you adhered to your espresso spending plan this week or wiped out your vehicle. At the point when you take a gander at it on paper or on-screen, you may be shocked at how these seemingly insignificant details add up.

Assuming it feels accommodating, allude back to this rundown when you find your considerations spiraling.

STAY PRESENT

Not prepared to focus on a reflection schedule? There are a lot of alternate ways of establishing yourself right now.

Be here at this point

The following are a couple of thoughts:

Turn off. Shut down your PC or telephone for an assigned measure of time every day, and invest that energy in a solitary action.

Eat carefully. Indulge yourself with one of your number one dinners. Attempt to track down the delight in each nibble, and truly center around how the food tastes, scents, and feels in your mouth.

Get outside. Go for a stroll outside, regardless of whether it's simply a fast lap around the block. Take stock of what you see en route, noticing any scents that drift by or sounds you hear.

CONSIDER DIFFERENT PERSPECTIVES

Some of the time, calming your contemplations requires venturing beyond your typical viewpoint. How you see the world is formed by your background, values, and suppositions. Envisioning things according to an alternate perspective can assist you with managing a portion of the clamor.

Write down a portion of the contemplations twirling around in your mind. Attempt to research how legitimate everyone is. For instance, perhaps you're fretting over an impending excursion since you simply know being a disaster is going. Yet, is that actually what will occur? What sort of confirmation do you need to back that up?

TAKE ACTIVITY

In some cases, you could go over similar contemplations more than once in light of the fact that you're not making any substantial moves about a specific circumstance.

Can't quit pondering somebody you begrudge? Rather than having it ruin your day, let your sentiments assist you with settling on better decisions.

Whenever you're visited by the green-peered beast, be proactive and write down ways you can approach arriving at your objectives. This will get you as far away from yourself as possible and channel your energy into making significant strides.

PRACTICE SELF-SYMPATHY

Harping on previous mishaps holds you back from giving up. Assuming that you're pummeling yourself over something you did keep going week, take a stab at pulling together on self-sympathy

Here are far to kick you off:

- Observe an unpleasant idea.

- Focus on the feelings and substantial reactions that emerge.

- Recognize that your sentiments are valid for you at the time.

- Take on an expression that addresses you, for example, "May I acknowledge myself as I am" or "I'm sufficient."

EMBRACE YOUR FEELINGS OF TREPIDATION

A few things will constantly be beyond your control. Figuring out how to acknowledge this can go quite far toward checking to overthink. One review from the 2018 Trusted Source demonstrates the way that tolerating negative considerations and fears can assist with working on mental wellbeing.

Obviously, this is more difficult than one might expect, and it will not come about pretty much by accident. Yet, search for little open doors where you can defy the circumstances you habitually stress over. Perhaps it's facing a bossy collaborator or requiring that independent road trip you've been longing for.

ASK FOR HELP

You don't need to go solo. Looking for outside help from a certified specialist can assist you with growing new instruments for managing your considerations and, surprisingly, having an impact on your outlook.

CHAPTER THREE

WHAT IS RUMINATION?

Has your head at any point been loaded up with one single idea, or a series of contemplations, that simply keep endlessly rehashing the same thing?

The course of ceaselessly contemplating similar considerations, which will generally be miserable or dim, is called rumination.

A propensity for rumination can be hazardous to your psychological well-being, as it can drag out or escalate melancholy as well as impede your capacity to think and deal with feelings. It might likewise make you feel confined and can, as a general rule, drive individuals away.

WHAT CAUSES RUMINATING?

Individuals ruminate for different reasons. As indicated by the American Psychological Association, a few normal explanations behind rumination include:

- A conviction that by ruminating, you'll acquire knowledge about your life or an issue
- Having a past filled with close to home or actual injury
- Confronting continuous stressors that can't be controlled

Ruminating is additionally normal in individuals who have specific character qualities, which incorporate hairsplitting, neuroticism, and an extreme spotlight on one's associations with others.

You could tend to exaggerate your associations with others such a lot that you'll make enormous individual penances to keep up with your connections, regardless of whether they're not working for you.

METHODS FOR ADDRESSING RUMINATING CONTEMPLATIONS

When you stall out in a ruminating figured cycle, it tends to be difficult to receive in return. In the event that you truly do enter a pattern of such considerations, it means a lot to stop them as fast as conceivable to keep them from turning out to be more serious.

As when a ball is moving downhill, it's simpler to stop the ruminating contemplations when they initially begin rolling and have less speed than when they've built up momentum over the long run.

Anyway, how might you prevent these over-the-top considerations from going through your head?

The following are 10 hints to attempt when you start to encounter a similar idea or set of considerations, whirling around your head:

DIVERT YOURSELF

At the point when you understand you're beginning to ruminate, finding an interruption can break your thinking cycle. Check out you, immediately pick another thing to do, and don't really think about it. Consider:

- Calling a companion or relative
- Finishing errands around your home
- Watching a film
- Drawing an image
- Perusing a book
- Strolling around your area

PLAN TO MAKE A MOVE

Rather than rehashing a similar negative idea, again and again, take that idea and make an arrangement to make a move to address it.

In your mind, frame each step you really want to take to resolve the issue or record it on a piece of paper. Be essentially as unambiguous as could be expected and reasonable with your assumptions.

Doing this will upset your rumination. It will likewise assist you with pushing ahead in the endeavor to get a negative thought out about your head unequivocally.

MAKE A MOVE

Whenever you've illustrated a game plan to address your ruminating contemplations, find one little way to resolve the issue. Allude to the arrangement you made to take care of the issue you've been fixating on.

Push ahead with each step gradually and steadily until your brain is reassured.

QUESTION YOUR CONSIDERATIONS

We frequently ruminate when we think we've committed a significant error or when something horrendous has happened to us that we feel liable for.

On the off chance that you begin ruminating on a disturbing idea, have a go at placing your redundant idea in context.

Contemplating your disturbing's thought process probably won't be precise but may assist you with halting ruminating on the grounds because the idea has neither rhyme nor reason.

CORRECT YOUR LIFE'S OBJECTIVES

Hairsplitting and unreasonable objective setting can prompt rumination. Assuming you put forth objectives that are unreasonable, you might begin to zero in on why and how you haven't arrived at an objective, or how you ought to have arrived at it.

Defining more practical objectives that you're equipped for accomplishing can lessen the dangers of overthinking your own decisions.

WORK ON UPGRADING YOUR CONFIDENCE

Many individuals who ruminate report troubles with confidence. Truth be told, the absence of confidence can be related to expanded rumination. It's additionally been connected with an expanded chance of misery.

Upgrade of confidence can be achieved in numerous ways. For example, expanding on existing qualities can add to a feeling of dominance, which can improve confidence.

Certain individuals might decide to chip away at the upgrade of confidence in psychotherapy. As you upgrade your confidence, self-viability may likewise be improved. You might observe that you're better ready to control rumination.

ATTEMPT CONTEMPLATION

Pondering can diminish rumination since it includes clearing your psyche to show up in a genuinely quiet state.

At the point when you end up with a rehashing circle of contemplations to you, search out a peaceful space. Plunk down, inhale profoundly, and center around only relaxing.

FIGURE OUT YOUR TRIGGERS

Each time you end up ruminating, give careful consideration to the circumstance you are in. This incorporates where you are, what season of the day it is, who's around you (on the off chance that anybody), and what you've been doing that day.

Creating ways of staying away from or dealing with these triggers can decrease your rumination.

CONVERSE WITH A COMPANION

Ruminating considerations can cause you to feel confined. Discussing your contemplations with a deal and an external viewpoint companion might assist with breaking the cycle.

Make certain to talk with a companion who can give you that point of view instead of ruminating with you.

ATTEMPT TREATMENT

On the off chance that your ruminating contemplations are assuming control over your life, you might need to think about treatment. A specialist can assist you with distinguishing why you're ruminating and how to resolve the issues at their center.

James C. Clever

CHAPTER FOUR

CONCLUSION

Ruminations include over-thinking or fixating on our sentiments, life-altering situations, pessimistic encounters, circumstances, or individuals. Ruminating contemplations are nosy and overpowering and frequently connected to antagonistic psychological wellness results, for example, nervousness, melancholy, post-horrendous pressure problem, dietary issues, etc.

At the point when you ruminate, you can't quit contemplating a pessimistic encounter or feelings. Infrequent ruminating considerations are normal, as everybody thinks about once in a while. You may unnecessarily ponder an impending distressing occasion like clinical intercession, significant execution, sports rivalry, or a last, most important test.

By the by, there is a distinction between pondering issues that can be tackled and ruminations about the things you have zero commands over in your life. Such ruminations are in many cases a piece of uneasiness and gloom issues.

Ruminating contemplations may likewise be set off by a new horrendous mishap, a particular stressor, or your character qualities like compulsiveness. Likewise, individuals with low confidence or self-perception issues are inclined to over-pondering their defects. At last, if you have a fear, you might ruminate on your feelings of dread when you need to confront them (for instance, an individual with a feeling of dread toward flying going via air).

In this way, when we are stressed, upset, or miserable, we will quite often over-think connections, sentiments, and valuable encounters.

However, certain individuals tend to overthink until they worry themselves. What's more, they fixate on nearly anything. Tenacious rumination might be an indication of a psychological well-being condition, so you might need to address your propensity to overthink everything with your PCP.

Ruminations are disastrous idea designs that can be unsafe to our mental and profound prosperity. We go after ruminations since they give a misguided feeling of command over our lives. In any case, as multitudinous things are outside of our reach or power, overthinking is frequently pointless, causing you to feel much more restless, befuddled, or troubled.

Nonetheless, if you have practiced the techniques discussed in this book, you would have come out successfully and quit overthinking everything in your life and recover certainty.

www.ingramcontent.com/pod-product-compliance
Lightning Source LLC
Chambersburg PA
CBHW060212260726
48658CB00005BA/2005